FERTILITY DIET COOKBOOK FOR WOMEN

20 Recipes to Improve Fertility and Boost Chances of Conception

Willie S. Harper

TABLE OF CONTENT

Introduction

Lily and David, a young couple, used to live in a peaceful neighbourhood hidden among the hills. Despite their best efforts, it didn't seem as though they would be able to have the kids they had always desired. When they unintentionally came upon an old cookbook in their attic one day, they were feeling lost and dissatisfied.

Out of curiosity, they wiped aside the torn pages and discovered a hidden gem: the Fertility Diet Cookbook for Women. Lily and David were so interested that they decided to embark on a culinary adventure to unravel the mysteries hidden inside these pages.

As they began their culinary journey focused on conception, they discovered the transformative power of food. With each perfectly prepared meal, they gave their bodies a symphony of fertility-enhancing ingredients. Their days were filled with hearty meals, meticulously prepared following the cookbook's instructions, as well as beautiful salads bursting with vitality.

After several months, much to Lily and David's delight, their expectations for a beautiful, healthy kid were realized. They realized that the cookbook's recipes had been more than just directions for preparing food; rather, they had been a lighthouse, guiding them toward their eagerly anticipated parenthood.

In addition to being delicious and nourishing, the recipes in this cookbook include a guide for naturally increasing fertility. Use these meals and the knowledge they offer as your compass to guide you toward your objectives.

Chapter 1: Breakfast Boosters

1.1 Berry Blast Smoothie

- 1 cup mixed berries (strawberries, blueberries, raspberries)
- 1 ripe banana
- 1 cup almond milk (or any milk of your choice)
- 1 tablespoon honey or maple syrup (optional)
- 1 tablespoon chia seeds
- 1/2 cup Greek yogurt
- Ice cubes (optional)

Instructions:

1. Wash the berries thoroughly and remove any stems or leaves.
2. In a blender, combine the mixed berries, banana, almond milk, honey or maple syrup (if desired), chia seeds, and Greek yogurt.
3. Blend on high speed until smooth and creamy.
4. If desired, add a few ice cubes and blend again for a chilled smoothie.
5. Pour the smoothie into a glass and serve immediately. Enjoy the refreshing and nutritious Berry Blast Smoothie!

Cook Time: 5 minutes

1.2 Green Goddess Omelette

- 3 large eggs
- 1/4 cup fresh spinach, chopped
- 2 tablespoons fresh parsley, chopped

- 1 tablespoon fresh basil, chopped
- 1 tablespoon fresh chives, chopped
- 1/4 cup grated mozzarella cheese (optional)
- Salt and pepper to taste
- 1 tablespoon olive oil

Instructions:

1. In a bowl, whisk the eggs until well beaten. Season with salt and pepper.
2. Heat olive oil in a non-stick skillet over medium heat.
3. Add the chopped spinach, parsley, basil, and chives to the skillet. Sauté for a minute until the spinach wilts.
4. Pour the beaten eggs into the skillet, spreading them evenly.
5. Sprinkle the grated mozzarella cheese (if using) over the eggs.
6. Cook the omelette for 2-3 minutes or until the edges are set.
7. Carefully fold the omelette in half using a spatula.
8. Cook for another minute until the cheese melts and the omelette is fully cooked.
9. Slide the omelette onto a plate and garnish with additional fresh herbs if desired.
10. Serve the Green Goddess Omelette hot and enjoy a flavorful and nutritious breakfast!

Cook Time: 10 minutes

1.3 Quinoa Breakfast Bowl

- 1/2 cup cooked quinoa
- 1/4 cup fresh berries (such as strawberries, blueberries, or raspberries)

- 1 tablespoon chopped nuts (almonds, walnuts, or pecans)
- 1 tablespoon honey or maple syrup
- 1/4 cup Greek yogurt
- 1 tablespoon chia seeds
- 1/2 teaspoon cinnamon (optional)
- Splash of milk (optional)

Instructions:

1. In a bowl, combine the cooked quinoa, fresh berries, and chopped nuts.
2. Drizzle honey or maple syrup over the quinoa mixture.
3. Add Greek yogurt on top of the quinoa.
4. Sprinkle chia seeds and cinnamon (if using) over the yogurt.
5. If desired, add a splash of milk to achieve the desired consistency.
6. Stir everything together gently until well combined.
7. Let the flavors meld for a few minutes.
8. Enjoy the Quinoa Breakfast Bowl as is or refrigerate for a refreshing chilled option.

Cook Time: 5 minutes

1.4 Avocado Toast with Poached Eggs

- 2 slices of whole grain bread
- 1 ripe avocado
- 2 large eggs
- Salt and pepper to taste
- Red pepper flakes (optional)
- Fresh cilantro or parsley, chopped (for garnish)

Instructions:

1. Toast the slices of whole grain bread to your desired level of crispness.
2. Cut the ripe avocado in half, remove the pit, and scoop the flesh into a bowl.
3. Mash the avocado with a fork until it reaches your desired consistency. Add salt and pepper to taste.
4. In a medium-sized pot, bring water to a gentle simmer. Crack the eggs into separate small bowls.
5. Carefully slide each egg into the simmering water, one at a time. Poach the eggs for about 3-4 minutes for a soft yolk.
6. While the eggs are poaching, spread the mashed avocado evenly onto the toasted bread slices.
7. Once the eggs are ready, use a slotted spoon to remove them from the water, allowing excess water to drain.
8. Place one poached egg on each avocado toast slice.
9. Sprinkle with salt, pepper, and red pepper flakes (if desired). Garnish with fresh cilantro or parsley.
10. Serve the Avocado Toast with Poached Eggs immediately for a delicious and satisfying breakfast.

Cook Time: 15 minutes

Chapter 2: Nourishing Lunches

2.1 Mediterranean Chickpea Salad

- 1 can chickpeas, drained and rinsed
- 1 cucumber, diced
- 1 cup cherry tomatoes, halved
- 1/2 red onion, thinly sliced
- 1/2 cup Kalamata olives, pitted and halved
- 1/4 cup fresh parsley, chopped
- 1/4 cup feta cheese, crumbled
- Juice of 1 lemon
- 2 tablespoons extra-virgin olive oil
- Salt and pepper to taste

Instructions:

1. In a large bowl, combine the chickpeas, cucumber, cherry tomatoes, red onion, Kalamata olives, and parsley.
2. In a small bowl, whisk together the lemon juice, olive oil, salt, and pepper.
3. Pour the dressing over the salad and toss gently to combine.
4. Sprinkle feta cheese over the top.
5. Refrigerate for at least 30 minutes to allow the flavors to meld.
6. Serve chilled as a refreshing and nutritious salad.

Cooking Time: 10 minutes

Preparation Time: 10 minutes

Total Time: 20 minutes

2.2 Grilled Salmon and Vegetable Skewers

- 2 salmon fillets, cut into cubes
- 1 zucchini, sliced
- 1 red bell pepper, cut into chunks
- 1 red onion, cut into chunks
- 8 cherry tomatoes
- 2 tablespoons olive oil
- 2 tablespoons lemon juice
- 2 cloves garlic, minced
- 1 teaspoon dried oregano
- Salt and pepper to taste

Instructions:

1. Preheat the grill to medium-high heat.
2. In a bowl, whisk together the olive oil, lemon juice, minced garlic, dried oregano, salt, and pepper.
3. Thread the salmon cubes, zucchini slices, red bell pepper chunks, red onion chunks, and cherry tomatoes onto skewers.
4. Brush the skewers with the marinade, making sure all the ingredients are coated.
5. Place the skewers on the preheated grill and cook for 4-5 minutes per side, or until the salmon is cooked through and the vegetables are tender.
6. Remove from the grill and let them rest for a few minutes before serving.

Cooking Time: 10 minutes

Preparation Time: 15 minutes

Total Time: 25 minutes

2.3 Spinach and Quinoa Stuffed Bell Peppers

- 4 bell peppers (any color), tops removed and seeds removed
- 1 cup cooked quinoa
- 1 cup baby spinach, chopped
- 1/2 cup cherry tomatoes, halved
- 1/2 cup feta cheese, crumbled
- 2 tablespoons pine nuts
- 2 tablespoons chopped fresh basil
- 1 tablespoon olive oil
- 1 clove garlic, minced
- Salt and pepper to taste

Instructions:

1. Preheat the oven to 375°F (190°C).
2. In a large bowl, combine cooked quinoa, chopped baby spinach, cherry tomatoes, feta cheese, pine nuts, chopped fresh basil, olive oil, minced garlic, salt, and pepper. Mix well.
3. Stuff each bell pepper with the quinoa and spinach mixture.
4. Place the stuffed bell peppers in a baking dish and cover with foil.
5. Bake for 30-35 minutes or until the bell peppers are tender.
6. Remove from the oven and let them cool for a few minutes before serving.

Cooking Time: 30-35 minutes

Preparation Time: 15 minutes

Total Time: 45-50 minutes

2.4 Lentil and Vegetable Soup

- 1 cup dried lentils, rinsed
- 1 onion, diced
- 2 carrots, diced
- 2 celery stalks, diced
- 2 cloves garlic, minced
- 4 cups vegetable broth
- 1 can diced tomatoes
- 1 teaspoon dried thyme
- 1 teaspoon ground cumin
- 1 bay leaf
- Salt and pepper to taste
- Fresh parsley for garnish (optional)

Instructions:

1. In a large pot, heat a tablespoon of olive oil over medium heat.
2. Add the diced onion, carrots, celery, and minced garlic. Sauté for 5 minutes or until the vegetables are slightly softened.
3. Add the rinsed lentils, vegetable broth, diced tomatoes, dried thyme, ground cumin, bay leaf, salt, and pepper to the pot. Stir well to combine.
4. Bring the soup to a boil, then reduce the heat to low and simmer for about 30-35 minutes or until the lentils are tender.
5. Remove the bay leaf and adjust the seasoning if needed.
6. Ladle the soup into bowls and garnish with fresh parsley, if desired.
7. Serve hot and enjoy the comforting flavors of this nourishing lentil and vegetable soup.

Cooking Time: 35-40 minutes

Preparation Time: 10 minutes

Total Time: 45-50 minutes

Chapter 3: Wholesome Snacks

3.1 Roasted Turmeric Chickpeas

- 2 cups canned chickpeas, drained and rinsed
- 1 tablespoon olive oil
- 1 teaspoon turmeric
- 1/2 teaspoon ground cumin
- 1/2 teaspoon paprika
- 1/4 teaspoon salt
- Freshly ground black pepper to taste

Instructions:

1. Preheat the oven to 400°F (200°C).
2. In a bowl, combine the chickpeas, olive oil, turmeric, cumin, paprika, salt, and black pepper. Toss until the chickpeas are evenly coated with the spices.
3. Spread the chickpeas in a single layer on a baking sheet.
4. Roast in the preheated oven for 25-30 minutes, or until the chickpeas are golden brown and crispy, shaking the pan occasionally to ensure even cooking.
5. Remove from the oven and let them cool slightly before serving.
6. Enjoy these flavorful and crunchy roasted turmeric chickpeas as a healthy snack or add them to salads for an extra boost of protein and fiber.

Cooktime: 25-30 minutes

3.2 Greek Yogurt Parfait with Berries

- 1 cup Greek yogurt
- 1/2 cup granola

- 1 cup mixed berries (strawberries, blueberries, raspberries)
- 2 tablespoons honey (optional)

Instructions:

1. In a glass or a bowl, start with a layer of Greek yogurt.
2. Add a layer of granola on top of the yogurt.
3. Arrange a portion of mixed berries over the granola.
4. Drizzle honey on top for added sweetness if desired.
5. Repeat the layers until all the ingredients are used, ending with a final sprinkle of berries on top.
6. Serve immediately and enjoy the delightful combination of creamy yogurt, crunchy granola, and juicy berries.

Cooktime: 5 minutes

3.3 Nutty Energy Bites

- 1 cup rolled oats
- 1/2 cup nut butter (such as almond or peanut butter)
- 1/4 cup honey or maple syrup
- 1/4 cup chopped nuts (such as almonds, walnuts, or cashews)
- 1/4 cup dried fruits (such as raisins, cranberries, or chopped dates)
- 1 tablespoon chia seeds (optional)
- 1 teaspoon vanilla extract
- Pinch of salt

Instructions:

1. In a large mixing bowl, combine all the ingredients and stir well until thoroughly combined.

2. Place the mixture in the refrigerator for about 30 minutes to allow it to firm up.
3. Once chilled, remove the mixture from the refrigerator and roll it into bite-sized balls using your hands.
4. Place the energy bites on a baking sheet lined with parchment paper.
5. Return the energy bites to the refrigerator for another 15-20 minutes to set.
6. Store the nutty energy bites in an airtight container in the refrigerator for up to a week.
7. Grab these nutritious and delicious bites whenever you need a quick energy boost or a satisfying snack on the go.

Cooktime: 1 hour (including chilling time)

3.4 Veggie Sushi Rolls

- 4 nori sheets
- 1 cup sushi rice, cooked and cooled
- 1 small carrot, julienned
- 1 small cucumber, julienned
- 1 small avocado, thinly sliced
- 1/4 cup pickled ginger
- 2 tablespoons soy sauce
- Wasabi and sesame seeds for serving (optional)

Instructions:

1. Place a nori sheet on a bamboo sushi mat or a clean kitchen towel.
2. Spread a thin layer of sushi rice evenly over the nori, leaving a 1-inch border at the top.

3. Arrange the julienned carrot, cucumber, and avocado slices in a horizontal line across the middle of the rice.
4. Starting from the bottom, tightly roll the nori sheet, using the sushi mat or towel to help you create a compact roll.
5. Wet the top border of the nori with water to seal the roll.
6. Repeat the process with the remaining nori sheets and ingredients.
7. Using a sharp knife, slice each sushi roll into bite-sized pieces.
8. Serve the veggie sushi rolls with pickled ginger, soy sauce, wasabi, and sesame seeds for dipping and added flavor.
9. Enjoy these homemade sushi rolls as a nutritious and satisfying meal or snack.

Cooktime: 30 minutes

Chapter 4: Nourishing Dinners

4.1 Quinoa and Black Bean Stuffed Bell Peppers

- 4 large bell peppers (any color)
- 1 cup cooked quinoa
- 1 cup black beans, rinsed and drained
- 1/2 cup corn kernels
- 1/2 cup diced tomatoes
- 1/2 cup shredded cheddar cheese
- 1/4 cup chopped fresh cilantro
- 1 teaspoon cumin
- 1/2 teaspoon chili powder
- Salt and pepper to taste

Instructions:

1. Preheat the oven to 375°F (190°C). Cut off the tops of the bell peppers and remove the seeds and membranes.
2. In a mixing bowl, combine cooked quinoa, black beans, corn kernels, diced tomatoes, shredded cheddar cheese, cilantro, cumin, chili powder, salt, and pepper. Stir well to combine.
3. Stuff each bell pepper with the quinoa and black bean mixture, packing it in tightly.
4. Place the stuffed bell peppers in a baking dish and cover with foil.
5. Bake for 25-30 minutes, or until the peppers are tender and the filling is heated through.
6. Remove the foil and bake for an additional 5 minutes to melt the cheese and lightly brown the tops.
7. Serve hot and garnish with extra cilantro, if desired.

Cook time: 35-40 minutes

4.2 Lemon Herb Baked Salmon

- 4 salmon fillets (about 6 ounces each)
- 2 lemons, sliced
- 4 sprigs of fresh dill
- 2 tablespoons olive oil
- 2 cloves garlic, minced
- 1 teaspoon dried thyme
- Salt and pepper to taste

Instructions:

1. Preheat the oven to 375°F (190°C). Line a baking sheet with parchment paper.
2. Place the salmon fillets on the prepared baking sheet. Season with salt and pepper.
3. In a small bowl, combine the olive oil, minced garlic, and dried thyme. Mix well.
4. Brush the olive oil mixture over the salmon fillets, coating them evenly.
5. Place lemon slices and fresh dill sprigs on top of each fillet.
6. Bake for 12-15 minutes, or until the salmon is cooked through and flakes easily with a fork.
7. Serve hot, garnished with extra lemon slices and dill sprigs.

Cook time: 12-15 minutes

4.3 Lentil Curry with Brown Rice

- 1 cup brown lentils, rinsed
- 1 onion, finely chopped
- 2 cloves garlic, minced

- 1 tablespoon curry powder
- 1 teaspoon turmeric
- 1 teaspoon cumin
- 1/2 teaspoon ginger powder
- 1/2 teaspoon paprika
- 1 can (14 ounces) coconut milk
- 1 cup vegetable broth
- 2 cups cooked brown rice
- Fresh cilantro for garnish
- Salt and pepper to taste

Instructions:

1. In a large pot, heat some oil over medium heat. Add the chopped onion and minced garlic, and sauté until softened and fragrant.
2. Add the curry powder, turmeric, cumin, ginger powder, and paprika to the pot. Stir well to coat the onions and garlic with the spices.
3. Add the rinsed lentils, coconut milk, and vegetable broth to the pot. Stir to combine all the ingredients.
4. Bring the mixture to a boil, then reduce the heat to low. Cover and simmer for 25-30 minutes, or until the lentils are tender.
5. Season with salt and pepper to taste.
6. Serve the lentil curry over cooked brown rice.
7. Garnish with fresh cilantro.

Cook time: 25-30 minutes

4.4 Grilled Chicken and Vegetable Stir-Fry

- 2 boneless, skinless chicken breasts, cut into thin strips

- 2 tablespoons soy sauce
- 2 tablespoons honey
- 1 tablespoon sesame oil
- 2 cloves garlic, minced
- 1 teaspoon grated fresh ginger
- 1 red bell pepper, thinly sliced
- 1 yellow bell pepper, thinly sliced
- 1 zucchini, sliced
- 1 cup broccoli florets
- 1 cup snap peas
- 1 tablespoon vegetable oil
- Salt and pepper to taste

Instructions:

1. In a small bowl, whisk together the soy sauce, honey, sesame oil, minced garlic, and grated ginger. Set aside.
2. Preheat a grill or grill pan over medium-high heat.
3. Season the chicken strips with salt and pepper.
4. Grill the chicken for 3-4 minutes per side, or until cooked through. Remove from the grill and set aside.
5. In a large skillet or wok, heat the vegetable oil over medium-high heat. Add the bell peppers, zucchini, broccoli, and snap peas. Stir-fry for 3-4 minutes, or until the vegetables are crisp-tender.
6. Return the grilled chicken to the skillet. Pour the soy sauce and honey mixture over the chicken and vegetables. Stir-fry for an additional 2-3 minutes, allowing the flavors to combine.
7. Remove from heat and serve hot over cooked rice or noodles.

Cook time: 20-25 minutes

Chapter 5: Sweet Treats

5.1 Dark Chocolate and Berry Parfait

- 1 cup Greek yogurt
- 2 tablespoons honey or maple syrup
- 1 teaspoon vanilla extract
- 1/4 cup dark chocolate chips
- 1 cup mixed berries (strawberries, blueberries, raspberries)
- Fresh mint leaves for garnish (optional)

Instructions:

1. In a bowl, combine Greek yogurt, honey or maple syrup, and vanilla extract. Mix well until smooth.
2. Melt the dark chocolate chips in a microwave-safe bowl, stirring every 15 seconds until fully melted.
3. Layer the parfait in glasses or bowls. Start with a spoonful of the yogurt mixture, followed by a drizzle of melted dark chocolate and a handful of mixed berries. Repeat the layers until the glasses or bowls are filled.
4. Finish with a dollop of the yogurt mixture on top and garnish with fresh mint leaves, if desired.
5. Serve immediately or refrigerate for 1-2 hours to allow flavors to meld. Enjoy this delightful and indulgent parfait!

Cook time: 10 minutes

5.2 Mango Coconut Chia Pudding

- 1/4 cup chia seeds
- 1 cup coconut milk

- 1 ripe mango, diced
- 2 tablespoons honey or agave syrup
- 1/4 teaspoon vanilla extract
- Shredded coconut for garnish (optional)

Instructions:

1. In a bowl, combine chia seeds and coconut milk. Stir well to prevent clumping. Let it sit for 5 minutes, then stir again.
2. In a blender or food processor, blend half of the diced mango until smooth. Add honey or agave syrup and vanilla extract to the mango puree and blend again.
3. In serving glasses or jars, layer the chia pudding and mango puree. Start with a spoonful of chia pudding, followed by a spoonful of mango puree. Repeat the layers until the glasses or jars are filled.
4. Top with the remaining diced mango and sprinkle with shredded coconut, if desired.
5. Refrigerate for at least 2 hours or overnight to allow the chia seeds to absorb the liquid and create a pudding-like texture.
6. Serve chilled and enjoy this tropical and nutritious chia pudding!

Cook time: 5 minutes + chilling time

5.3 Blueberry Almond Flour Muffins

- 2 cups almond flour
- 1/4 cup coconut flour
- 1/2 teaspoon baking soda
- 1/4 teaspoon salt
- 3 eggs

- 1/4 cup honey or maple syrup
- 1/4 cup melted coconut oil
- 1 teaspoon vanilla extract
- 1 cup fresh blueberries

Instructions:

1. Preheat the oven to 350°F (175°C) and line a muffin tin with paper liners.
2. In a large bowl, whisk together almond flour, coconut flour, baking soda, and salt.
3. In a separate bowl, beat the eggs. Add honey or maple syrup, melted coconut oil, and vanilla extract. Mix well.
4. Pour the wet ingredients into the dry ingredients and stir until fully combined.
5. Gently fold in the fresh blueberries.
6. Spoon the batter into the prepared muffin tin, filling each cup about 3/4 full.
7. Bake for 20-25 minutes or until a toothpick inserted into the center of a muffin comes out clean.
8. Allow the muffins to cool in the tin for 5 minutes, then transfer them to a wire rack to cool completely.
9. Enjoy these moist and flavorful blueberry almond flour muffins as a nutritious breakfast or snack!

Cook time: 20-25 minutes

5.4 Banana Walnut Bread

- 2 ripe bananas, mashed
- 1/4 cup melted coconut oil or unsalted butter
- 1/2 cup honey or maple syrup
- 2 eggs
- 1 teaspoon vanilla extract

- 1 3/4 cups almond flour
- 1/4 cup coconut flour
- 1 teaspoon baking soda
- 1/2 teaspoon salt
- 1/2 cup chopped walnuts

Instructions:

1. Preheat the oven to 350°F (175°C) and grease a loaf pan with coconut oil or butter.
2. In a large bowl, combine mashed bananas, melted coconut oil or butter, honey or maple syrup, eggs, and vanilla extract. Mix well.
3. In a separate bowl, whisk together almond flour, coconut flour, baking soda, and salt.
4. Gradually add the dry ingredients to the wet ingredients, stirring until just combined.
5. Fold in the chopped walnuts.
6. Pour the batter into the prepared loaf pan and smooth the top with a spatula.
7. Bake for 50-60 minutes or until a toothpick inserted into the center of the bread comes out clean.
8. Allow the bread to cool in the pan for 10 minutes, then transfer it to a wire rack to cool completely before slicing.
9. Slice and savor each delicious bite of this moist and nutty banana walnut bread!

Cook time: 50-60 minutes

Conclusion

Congratulations on completing the gastronomic journey of The Fertility Diet Cookbook for Women! You've already taken steps to improve your diet and naturally increase your fertility. By including these delicious and nutrient-dense meals into your routine, you've taken an active step toward establishing a healthy lifestyle.

Through this recipe, you've learned the crucial connection between nutrition and fertility. Each recipe has been carefully designed to provide you with the vitamins, minerals, and nutrients you need to promote the health of your reproductive organs. These recipes have given you a wide range of options to make your meals interesting and enjoyable, ranging from energizing breakfasts to substantial lunches and dinners.

Remember that this cookbook is more than a collection of dishes; it is a manual for a whole approach to fertility. A healthy lifestyle that includes regular exercise, stress management, and self-care is encouraged for you to adopt. By developing these practices, you empower yourself to control your reproductive process.

As you continue, keep studying more about the connection between nutrition and fertility. Try out different ingredient combinations, make the recipes your own, and trust your instincts. Stay in touch with your body and pay attention to its unique needs.

As you begin your parenthood journey, I wish you luck, strength, and bravery. As you set out on the amazing and life-altering journey of creating a family, I hope that this cookbook will be an invaluable resource and your traveling companion.

Remember that you have the power to nurture and preserve your fertility. Happy cooking and best wishes for a great and successful future!